7-MINUTE
CORE
EXERCISES

for Seniors Over 50

Easy-to-Follow Daily Routine to Build Confidence and Improve Balance and Mobility | 30-Day Beginner, Intermediate & Advanced Challenge to Improve Posture

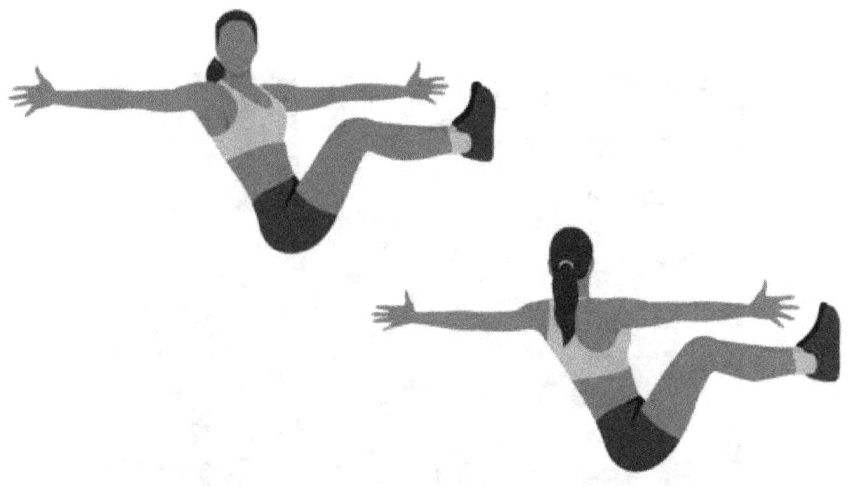

ERIC A. RANDELL

COPYRIGHT

No part of this book may be reproduced in written, electronic, recording, or photocopying without the permission of the publisher or author. The exception would be in the case of brief quotations embodied in the critical articles or reviews and pages where permission is specifically granted by the publisher or author.
Although every precaution has been taken to verify the accuracy of the information contained herein, the author and publisher assume responsibility for any errors or omissions. No liability is assumed for damages that may result from the use of the information contained within.
All Right Reserved©2024

SCAN HERE FOR MORE BOOKS FROM ME

ERIC A. RANDELL

TABLE OF CONTENTS

ERIC A. RANDELL

INTRODUCTION

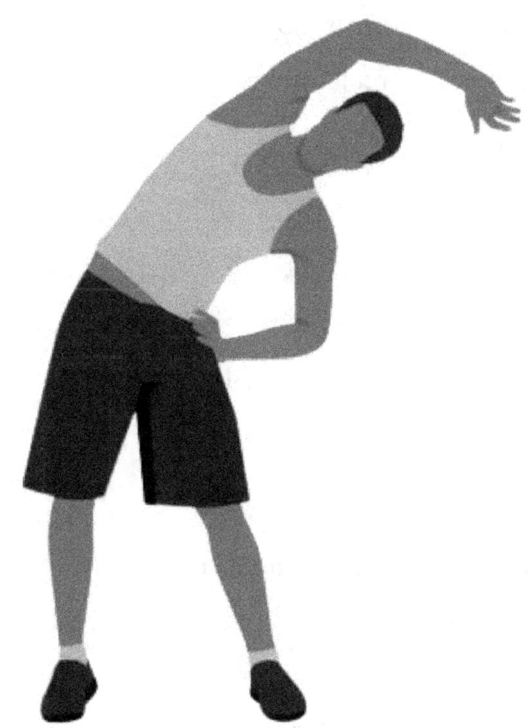

Welcome to "7-Minute Core Exercises for Seniors Over 50," a comprehensive and practical resource designed to empower adults over 50 with the knowledge and tools to enhance their overall fitness and well-being. In this fast-paced world, where time is a precious commodity, we understand the challenges of maintaining a healthy lifestyle while juggling numerous responsibilities. That's why we've crafted this book specifically for you – to help you prioritize your core strength and invest just seven minutes a day towards a stronger, healthier you.

Why do you need this book? As we age, our bodies undergo natural changes, often accompanied by a decline in core strength. This reduction can lead to a host of issues, such as decreased balance, stability, and flexibility. Everyday activities that were once effortless may become more challenging, limiting our independence and quality of life. But fear not! This book is your roadmap to revitalizing your core muscles and reclaiming your vitality.

Within these pages, you'll discover a treasure trove of simple yet effective exercises meticulously curated for adults over 50. Our workout routines are intelligently designed to target key muscle groups, including your abs, obliques, lower back, hips, and overall stability. Whether you're a fitness enthusiast looking to maintain your active lifestyle or someone who's just starting their fitness journey, there's something for everyone in this book.

What sets this book apart is our commitment to your safety and success. We understand that as we age, we require exercises that are gentle on the joints, mindful of previous injuries, and adaptable to individual fitness levels. That's why we've included expert tips and modifications, ensuring that each exercise can be tailored to your unique capabilities and goals. You'll find clear instructions, accompanied by illustrations, guiding you through proper form and technique, so you can exercise with confidence.

But this book is more than just the compilation of exercises—it's a holistic approach to well-being. We delve into the importance of warm-up and stretching, helping you prepare your body for the workout ahead. Moreover, we offer guidance on integrating core workouts into your weekly routine, providing sample schedules and tips for staying motivated.

By dedicating just seven minutes of your day to these core exercises, you'll embark on a transformative journey towards a stronger, more balanced you. As you progress, you'll witness the positive ripple effects in your daily life – increased stability, improved posture, enhanced performance in other physical activities, and a newfound sense of confidence.

7-Minute Core Exercises for Seniors Over 50 is your steadfast companion, supporting you every step of the way. It's time to prioritize your core strength, reclaim your vitality, and embrace a healthier, more active lifestyle. Are you ready to embark on this empowering journey? Let's strengthen your core and unlock your full potential!

THE IMPORTANCE OF CORE EXERCISES

Core strength is a fundamental aspect of our overall physical well-being, playing a pivotal role in our daily lives. It encompasses the muscles in our abdomen, back, and pelvis, providing stability, balance, and mobility to our bodies. But why does core strength matter? Let's delve into the importance of cultivating a strong core and understand its wide-ranging benefits.

1. **Enhances Posture:** A strong core helps maintain proper alignment and posture, reducing the strain on our back and spine. It acts as a stabilizer, preventing slouching and promoting an upright position. By improving our posture, we alleviate stress on our joints, decrease the risk of injuries, and enhance overall body mechanics.

2. **Supports Daily Activities:** Core strength is essential for performing everyday tasks, such as lifting, bending, twisting, and reaching. Whether we're carrying groceries, gardening, or simply getting up from a chair, a strong core provides the necessary stability and strength to execute these movements efficiently and with reduced risk of strain or injury.

3. **Enhances Balance and Stability:** As we age, maintaining balance becomes increasingly important. A strong core helps improve balance and stability, reducing the likelihood of falls and injuries. By strengthening the core muscles, we enhance our body's ability to react and stabilize itself in various situations, promoting confidence and independence in daily activities.

4. Boosts Athletic Performance: No matter what physical activities we engage in, a strong core is a game-changer. From running and cycling to playing sports or practicing yoga, a stable core enables efficient movement, transfers power between the upper and lower body, and enhances overall athletic performance. It serves as the foundation for generating strength, speed, and agility.

5. Alleviates Back Pain: One of the most common reasons people seek medical attention is back pain. A weak core often contributes to back pain and discomfort. Strengthening the core muscles can help alleviate and prevent such issues by providing support to the spine, improving spinal alignment, and reducing the strain on the back.

6. Improves Breathing and Digestion: The core plays a crucial role in supporting our respiratory and digestive systems. By strengthening the core muscles, we enhance diaphragmatic breathing, allowing for deeper breaths and increased oxygen intake. Additionally, a strong core aids in promoting healthy digestion and optimal functioning of the abdominal organs.

7. Enhances Overall Functional Fitness: A strong core forms the foundation for functional fitness. It facilitates coordinated movement, improves coordination between different muscle groups, and enables efficient energy transfer. Whether we're performing day-to-day activities or pursuing specific fitness goals, a strong core enhances our overall functional fitness, making tasks feel easier and more enjoyable.

Cultivating a strong core is not only about physical strength but also about improving our overall quality of life. It empowers us to move with ease, reduces the risk of injuries, and enhances our ability to engage in activities that bring us joy and fulfillment. By dedicating time and effort to core strengthening exercises, we invest in our long-term well-being, promoting a healthier, more active lifestyle.

ITEMS NEEDED FOR THE CORE EXERCISES

1. Exercise Mat: A comfortable, non-slip exercise mat will provide cushioning and support for exercises like planks, bridges, and crunches.

2. Stability Ball: A stability ball can be used for exercises such as stability ball crunches and seated Russian twists to improve balance and core strength.

3. Light Dumbbells: Optional light dumbbells can be used for exercises like woodchoppers and Russian twists to add resistance and challenge the muscles.

4. Resistance Bands: Resistance bands can be used for exercises like seated leg lifts and side-lying leg lifts to provide resistance and strengthen the muscles.

5. **Chair:** A stable chair can be used for exercises like seated leg lifts and chair sit-ups to assist with balance and support.

6. **Yoga Blocks:** Yoga blocks can be used for exercises like boat pose and side bends to aid in stability and alignment.

7. **Towel:** A small towel can be used as support for exercises like boat pose and seated leg lifts to maintain proper form and comfort.

GENERAL INSTRUCTIONS AND PRECAUTIONS TO ENSURE SAFETY

When engaging in any fitness regimen, especially as a senior over 50, safety is of utmost importance. Here are some key precautions and measures to ensure a safe and successful exercise journey:

Consult a Healthcare Provider: Before starting any exercise program, it's essential to consult with your healthcare provider. They can provide valuable guidance based on your individual health status and any existing medical conditions, and offer tailored recommendations to support your safety and well-being.

Appropriate Warm-up and Cool-down: Begin every exercise session with a proper warm-up to gradually increase blood flow to the muscles and prepare your body for physical activity. Likewise, end your workout with a thorough cool-down to reduce muscle tension and promote flexibility. Both the warm-up and cool-down phases play a significant role in preventing injuries.

Listen to Your Body: Pay close attention to your body's signals during exercise. If you experience unusual pain, dizziness, or shortness of breath, it's important to stop immediately and seek assistance. Understanding your body's limits and responding to its cues can help prevent overexertion and potential injuries.

Proper Form and Technique: Emphasize maintaining proper form and technique when performing exercises. This includes maintaining good posture, executing movements with control, and avoiding sudden, jerky motions that may strain muscles or joints.

Using the correct form also enhances the effectiveness of the exercise and reduces the risk of injury.

Stay Hydrated: Ensure you remain adequately hydrated before, during, and after exercising, as dehydration can adversely affect your performance and health. Keep a water bottle nearby and drink water regularly to maintain proper hydration levels.

Comfortable and Safe Environment: Create a safe and clear space for your exercise routine, free from obstacles or tripping hazards. Additionally, ensure that any equipment used is in good condition and is used in a safe and appropriate manner.

Regular Health Check-ups: As you progress on your exercise journey, schedule regular check-ups with your healthcare provider to monitor your overall health and any changes in your physical condition. This can help in adjusting your exercise routine as needed.

ANSWERS TO MYTHS ABOUT CORE AND STRENGTH EXERCISES FOR SENIORS

1. Myth: ***Seniors should avoid strength training because it can lead to injury.***

Answer: This is not true. In fact, strength training can actually help prevent injury in seniors by improving muscle mass, bone density, and balance, reducing the risk of falls and fractures.

2. Myth: ***Seniors cannot build muscle or strength.***

Answer: While it may be more challenging for seniors to build muscle and strength compared to younger individuals, research shows that with proper training and nutrition, seniors can still make significant improvements in muscle mass and strength.

3. Myth: ***Strength training is only for younger people.***

Answer: Strength training is beneficial for individuals of all ages, including seniors. It can help maintain independence, improve functional abilities, and enhance overall quality of life.

4. Myth: *Seniors should only focus on cardio exercise.*

Answer: While cardio exercise is important for heart health, incorporating strength training into a senior's fitness routine is essential for maintaining muscle mass, bone density, and overall strength and mobility.

5. Myth: *Seniors should only use light weights for strength training.*

Answer: Research suggests that seniors can use heavier weights with proper supervision and technique. Using heavier weights can help stimulate muscle growth and strength improvements.

6. Myth: *Strength training will make seniors bulky.*

Answer: Seniors do not have the same hormone levels as younger individuals, so they are less likely to experience significant muscle bulk. Strength training for seniors is more focused on maintaining functional strength and mobility.

7. Myth: *Seniors with arthritis should avoid strength training.*

Answer: Many studies have shown that strength training can actually help alleviate arthritis symptoms by improving joint stability, reducing pain, and improving overall function and mobility.

8. Myth: *Seniors will experience a decline in strength no matter what they do.*

Answer: While muscle mass and strength do naturally decline with age, research has shown that consistent strength training can help minimize this decline and even lead to strength improvements.

9. Myth: *Seniors should not lift weights overhead.*

Answer: Lifting weights overhead can actually help improve shoulder strength and mobility, as long as it is done with proper technique and progression.

10. Myth: *Strength training is not safe for seniors with chronic conditions.*

Answer: Many chronic conditions, such as diabetes, heart disease, and osteoporosis, can actually benefit from strength training. It can help improve insulin sensitivity, cardiovascular health, and bone density, among other benefits. As always, it is important for seniors with chronic conditions to consult with their healthcare provider before starting a new exercise program.

LET'S BEGIN NOW

PLANK

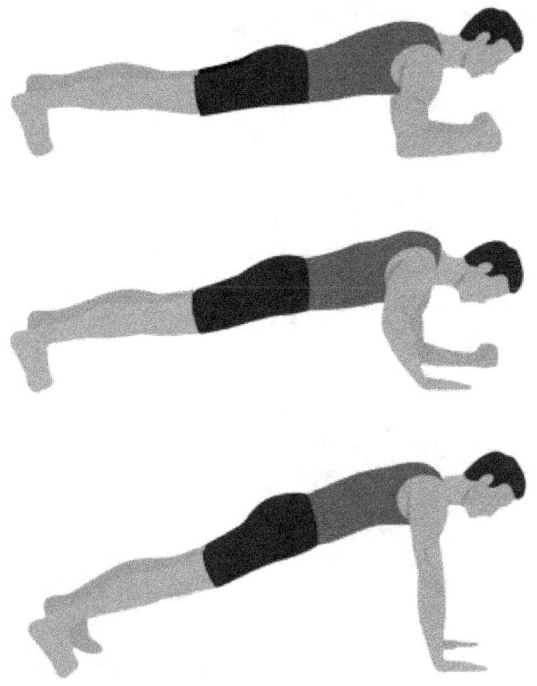

INSTRUCTIONS:

➤ Start by getting into a push-up position, with your hands directly under your shoulders and your body forming a straight line from your head to your heels.

➤ Engage your core muscles and hold this position for 20-30 seconds, making sure to keep your hips level and not allowing them to sag or hike up.

➤ As you build strength, increase the duration of the hold to 45-60 seconds.

➤ For seniors over 50 years, it is recommended to start with 3 sets of 20-30 seconds hold, gradually increasing to 3 sets of 45-60 seconds as strength and endurance improve.

RUSSIAN TWISTS

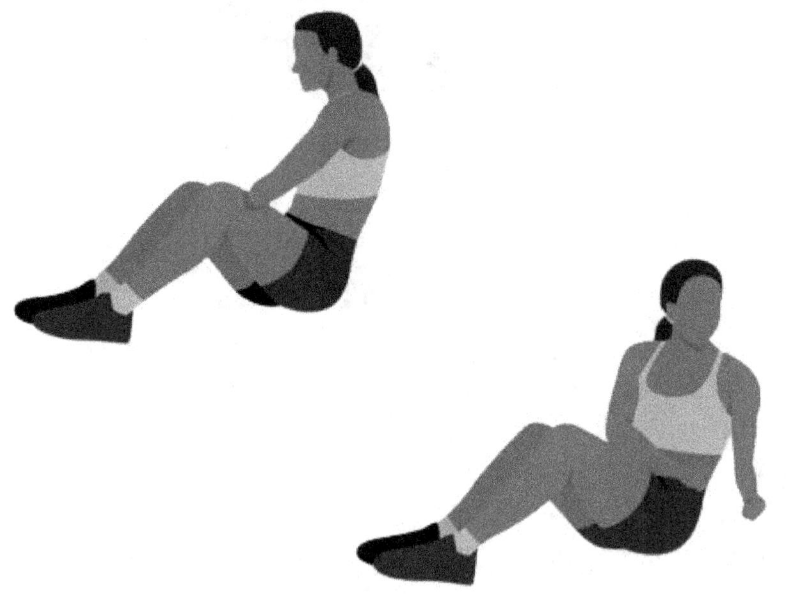

INSTRUCTIONS:

➤ Begin this exercise by sitting on the floor with your knees bent and your feet flat. Lean back slightly forming a V-shape with your thighs.

➤ Clasp your hands in front of you and raise them to chest level, keeping your arms straight.

- ➤ Engage your core and twist your torso to the right, bringing your hands beside your right hip. Then twist to the left.
- ➤ Start with 10-15 repetitions, gradually increasing to 20-25 as strength improves. Hold each twist for 20-30 seconds.

BICYCLE CRUNCHES

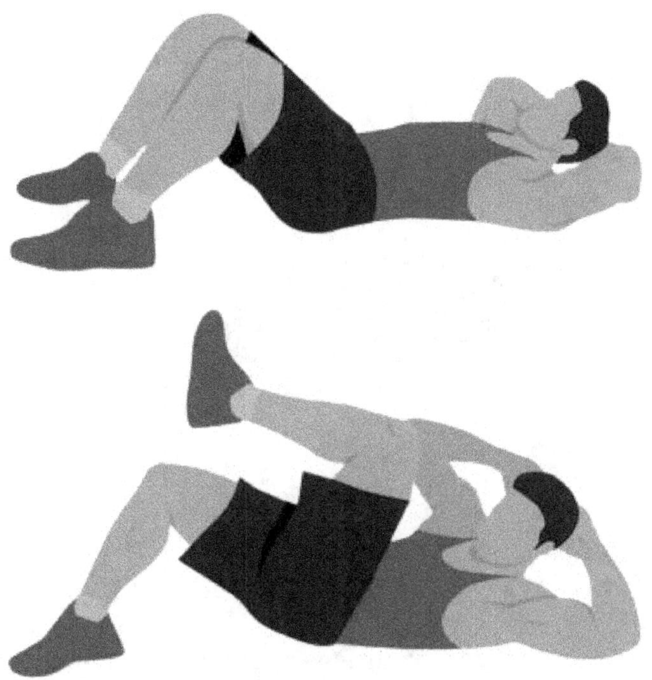

INSTRUCTIONS:

- ➤ Lie on your back with your hands behind your head, legs raised, and knees bent at a 90-degree angle.

> Bring your right elbow and left knee towards each other while straightening out your right leg.

> Alternate to bring your left elbow and right knee together while straightening your left leg.

> Aim for 10-15 repetitions to start, increasing to 20-25 as strength improves.

SIDE PLANK

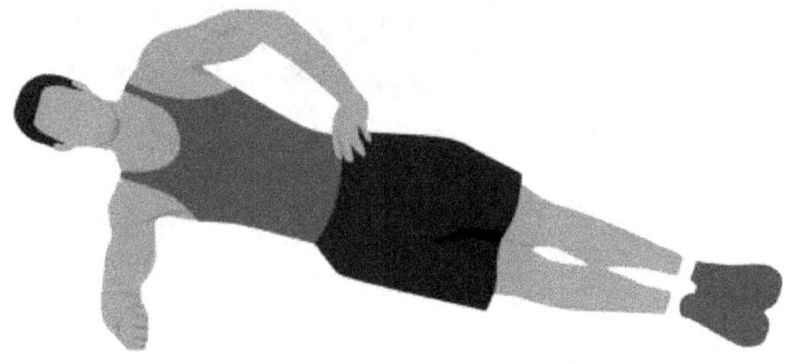

INSTRUCTIONS:

> Lie on your side with your legs straight and prop your body up on your forearm, keeping your body in a straight line.

> Hold the position for 20-30 seconds to start, gradually increasing to 45-60 seconds. Repeat on the other side.

DEAD BUG

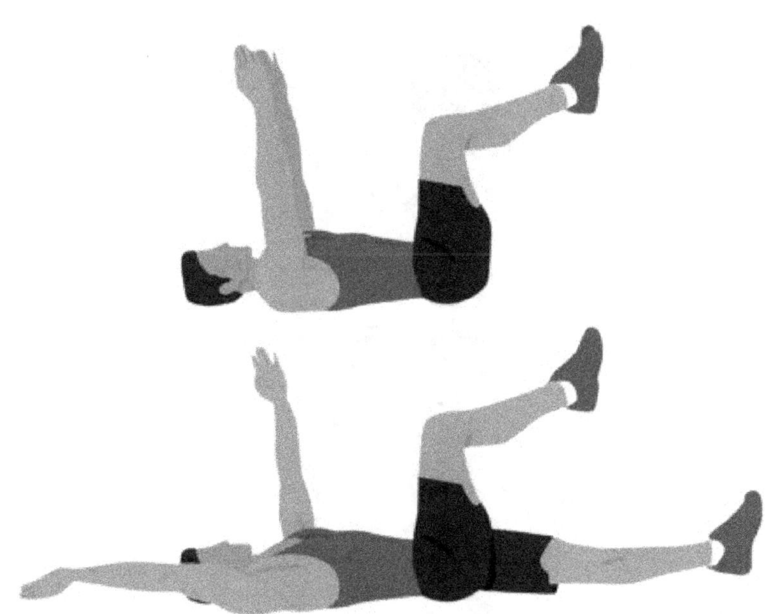

INSTRUCTIONS:

➢ Lie on your back with knees bent, shins parallel to the floor, and arms extended straight up toward the ceiling.

➢ Lower your right arm and left leg toward the floor, keeping your lower back pressed to the ground.

➢ Now, return to the starting/initial position and then lower your left arm and right leg.

➢ Aim for 10-12 repetitions on each side to start, gradually increasing to 15-20 repetitions.

BIRD DOG

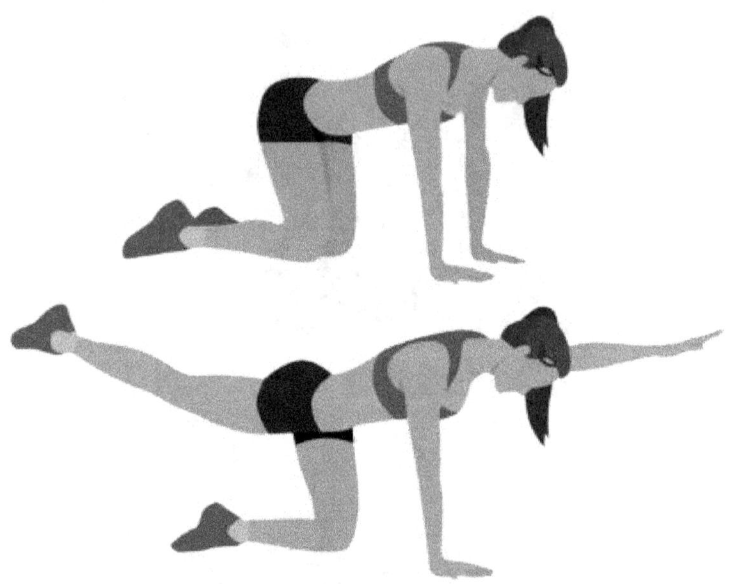

INSTRUCTIONS:

➤ Start on all fours with your hands aligned under shoulders and knees under hips.

➤ Lift your right arm and left leg, extending them straight out from your body. Hold for a few seconds.

➤ Return to the starting position and then lift your left arm and right leg.

➤ Aim for 10-12 repetitions on each side, gradually increasing to 15-20 repetitions.

SUPERMAN

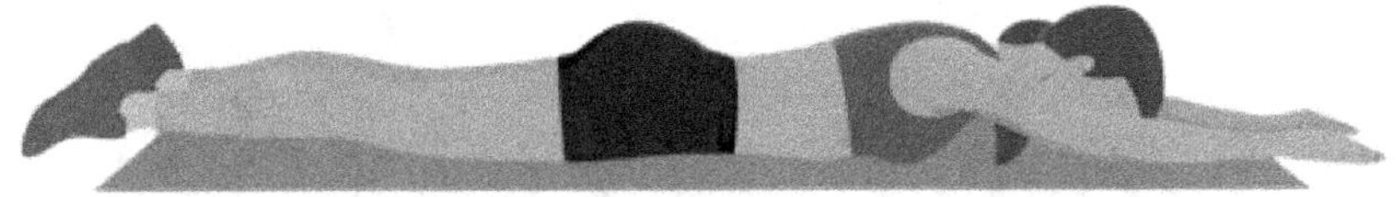

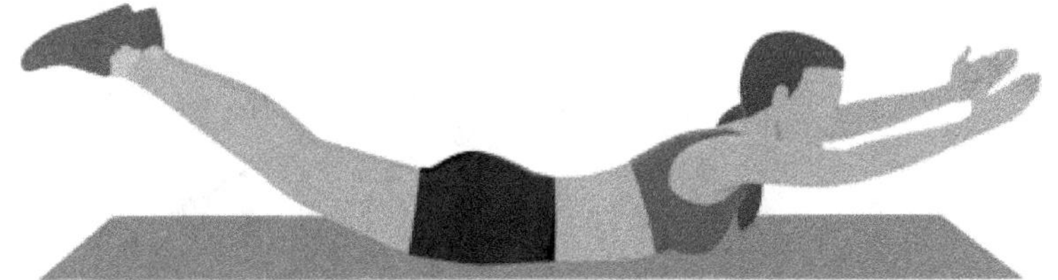

INSTRUCTIONS:

➤ Start by lying face down with your arms extended in front of you.

➤ Gently and carefully lift your arms, chest, and legs off the ground simultaneously, squeezing your glutes and lower back muscles.

➤ Hold for 10-15 seconds, and aim for 5-8 repetitions.

TUCK CRUNCHES

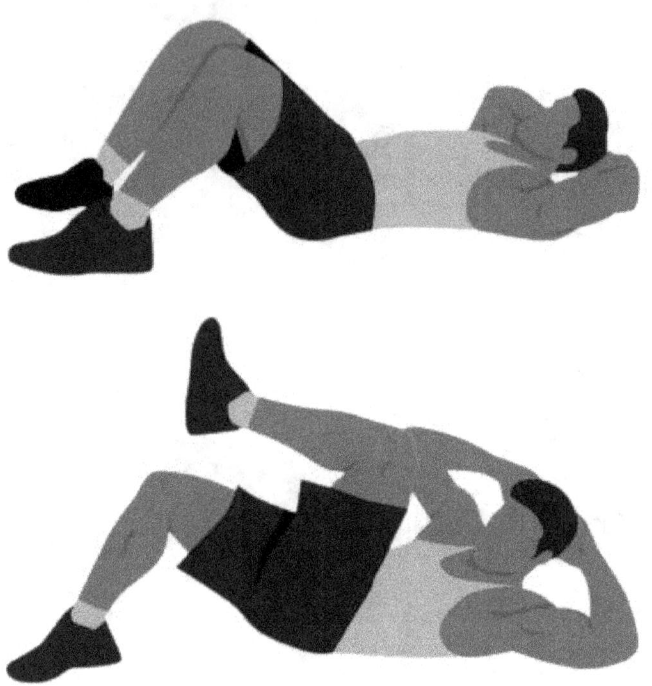

INSTRUCTIONS:

➢ Lie down with your knees bent and feet flat on the floor.

➢ Perform a crunch, bringing your knees towards your chest as you lift your shoulder blades off the ground.

➢ Aim for 10-15 repetitions, gradually increasing to 20-25 as strength improves.

LEG RAISES

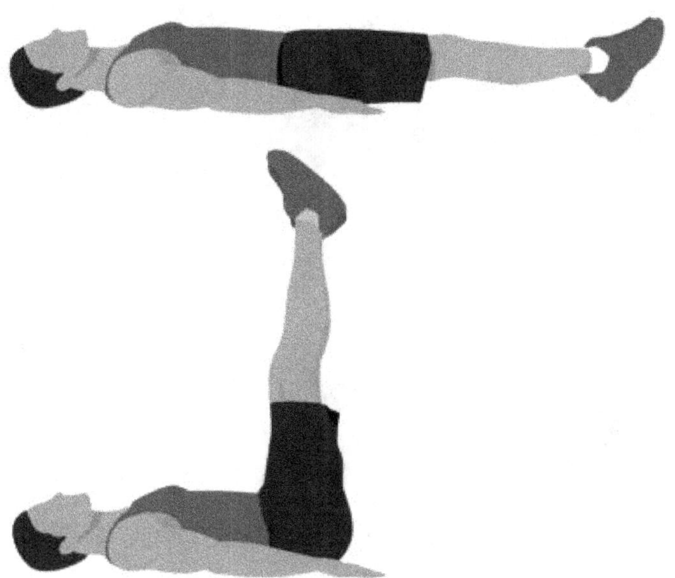

INSTRUCTIONS:

➢ Lie on your back with legs straight and hands under your hips for support.

➢ Lift both legs off the ground, keeping them straight.

➢ Lower them back down without touching the ground.

➢ Aim for 10-12 repetitions, gradually increasing to 15-20 as strength improves.

FLUTTER KICKS

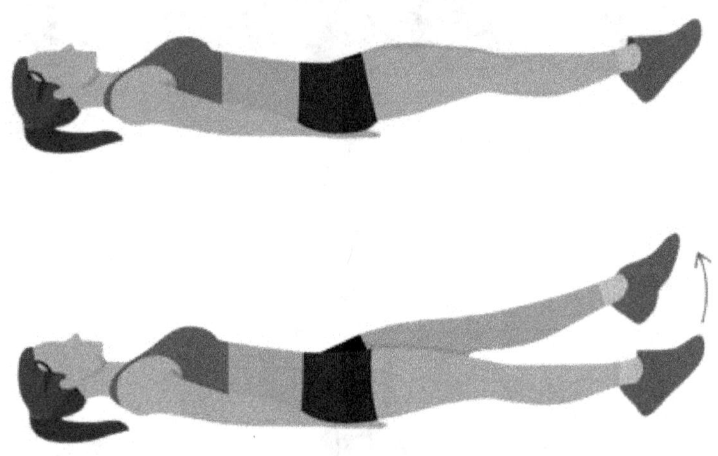

INSTRUCTIONS:

➤ Start by lying on your back with your legs straight.

➤ Lift your legs a few inches off the ground and alternate kicking up and down in a fluttering motion.

➤ Aim for 20-30 seconds, gradually increasing to 45-60 seconds.

SCISSOR KICKS

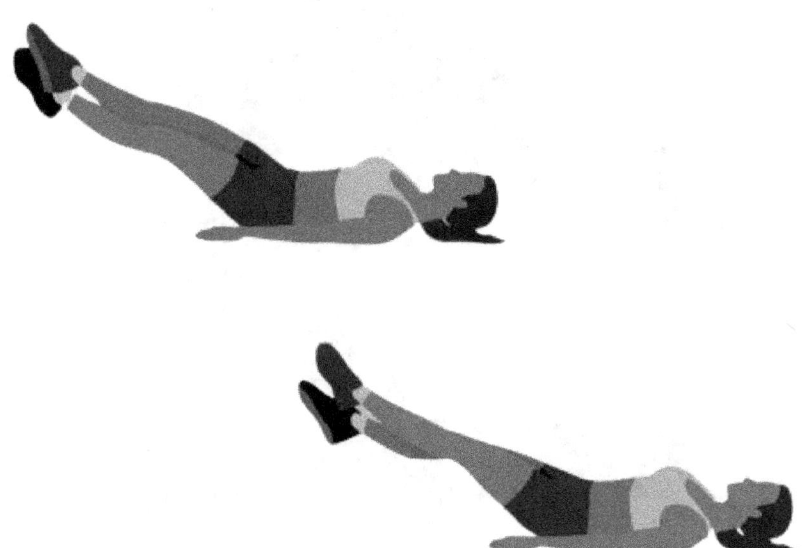

INSTRUCTIONS:

➢ Start this exercise by lying on your back with your legs straight.

➢ Next, gently lift your legs a few inches off the ground, then cross one leg over the other, alternating back and forth in a scissoring motion.

➢ Aim for 20-30 seconds, gradually increasing to 45-60 seconds.

BRIDGE

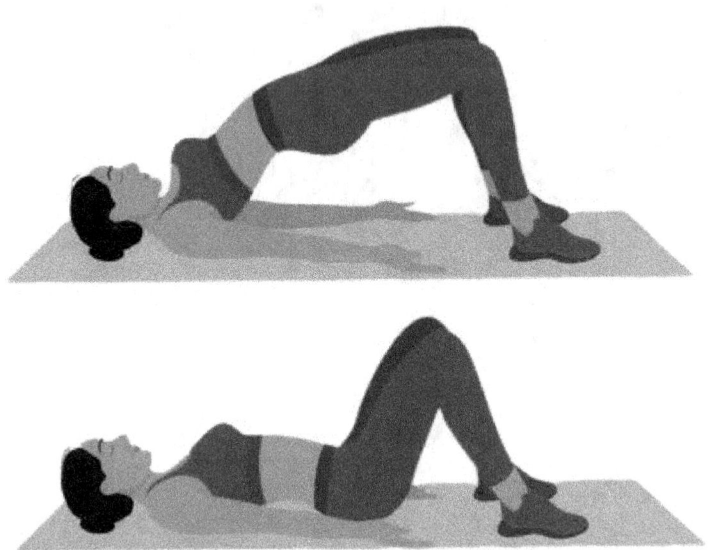

INSTRUCTIONS:

➢ Start this exercise by lying on your back with your knees bent and feet flat on the floor.

➢ Next, gently lift your hips towards the ceiling, creating a straight line from shoulders to knees.

➢ Hold for 20-30 seconds to start, gradually increasing to 45-60 seconds.

SIT-UPS

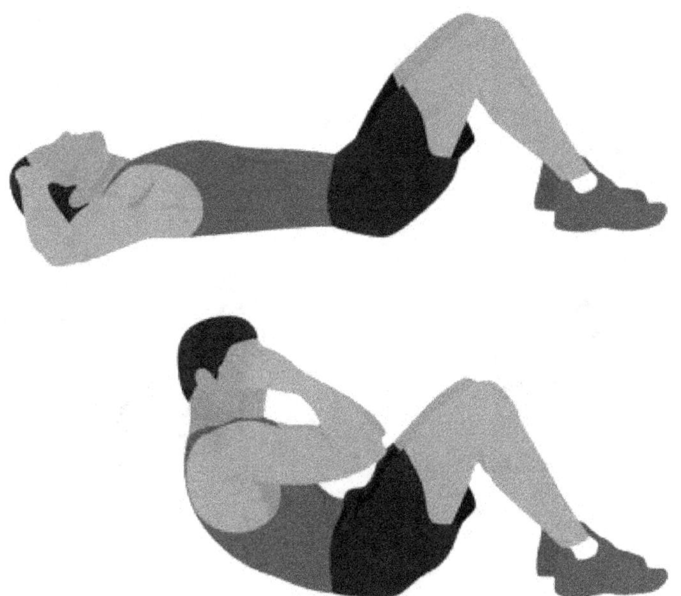

INSTRUCTIONS:

➢ Start this exercise by lying on your back with your knees bent and feet flat on the floor.

➢ Place your hands behind your head and engage your core to lift your upper body off the ground.

➢ Aim for 10-15 repetitions to start, gradually increasing to 20-25 as strength improves.

REVERSE CRUNCHES

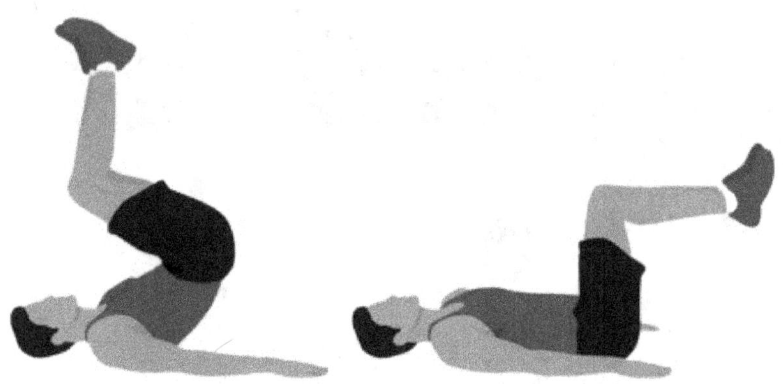

INSTRUCTIONS:

➢ Start this exercise by lying on your back with your knees bent and feet flat on the floor.

➢ Lift your legs, bring your knees towards your chest and lift your hips off the ground.

➢ Aim for 10-12 repetitions to start, gradually increasing to 15-20 as strength improves.

BOAT POSE

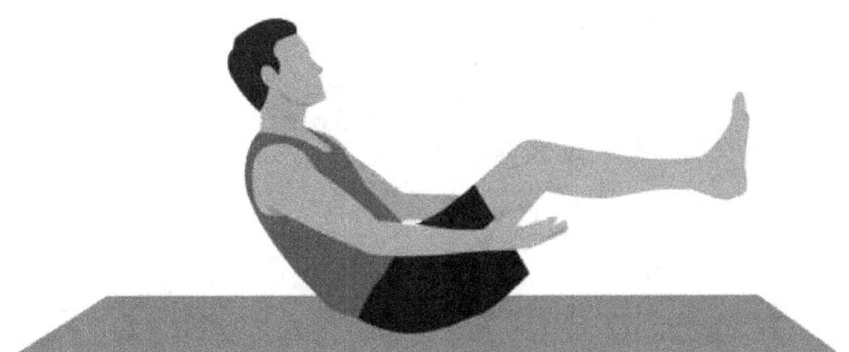

INSTRUCTIONS:

> Start this boat pose by sitting on the floor with your knees bent and feet flat.

> Lean back slightly and lift your feet off the ground, straightening your legs to form a V-shape with your body.

> Hold for 20-30 seconds to start, gradually increasing to 45-60 seconds.

MOUNTAIN CLIMBERS

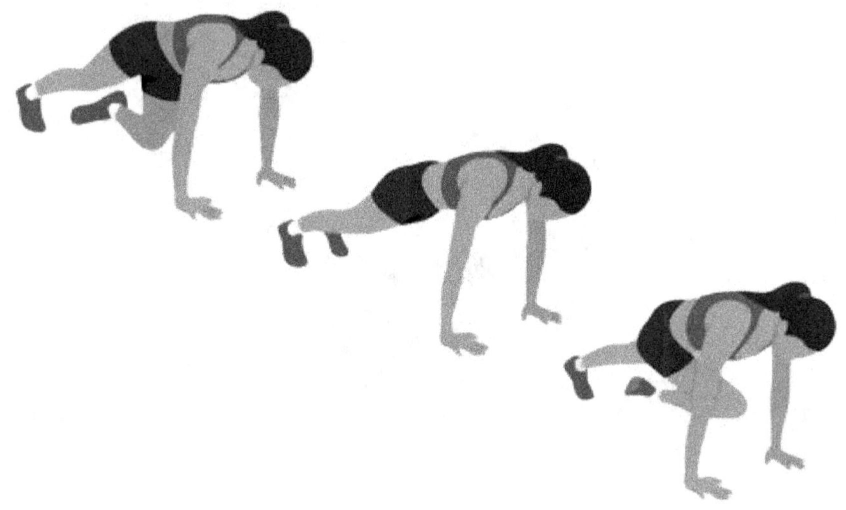

INSTRUCTIONS:

➢ Begin this exercise in a plank position with your hands directly under your shoulders.

➢ Next, bring one knee towards your chest, then switch legs in a running motion.

➢ Aim for 20-30 seconds, gradually increasing to 45-60 seconds.

V-SIT

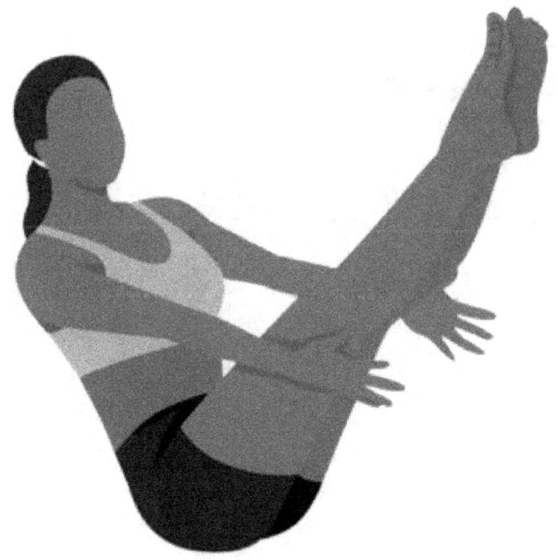

INSTRUCTIONS:

➤ Sit on the floor with your legs extended in front of you.

➤ Lean back slightly and lift your legs and upper body, reaching your hands towards your feet to form a V-shape.

➤ Hold for 20-30 seconds to start, gradually increasing to 45-60 seconds.

STABILITY BALL CRUNCHES

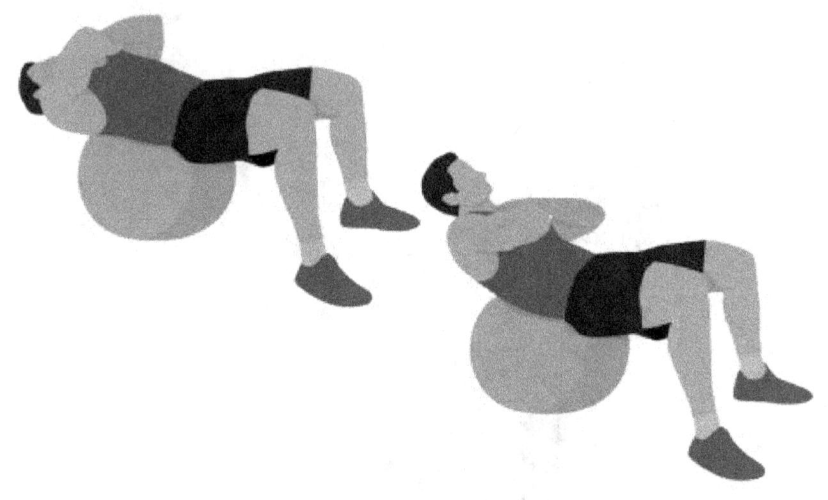

INSTRUCTIONS:

➢ Start this exercise by sitting on a stability ball with your feet flat on the floor and knees bent.

➢ Cross your arms over your chest and engage your core to perform a crunch.

➢ Aim for 10-15 repetitions to start, gradually increasing to 20-25 as strength improves.

WALKING PLANKS

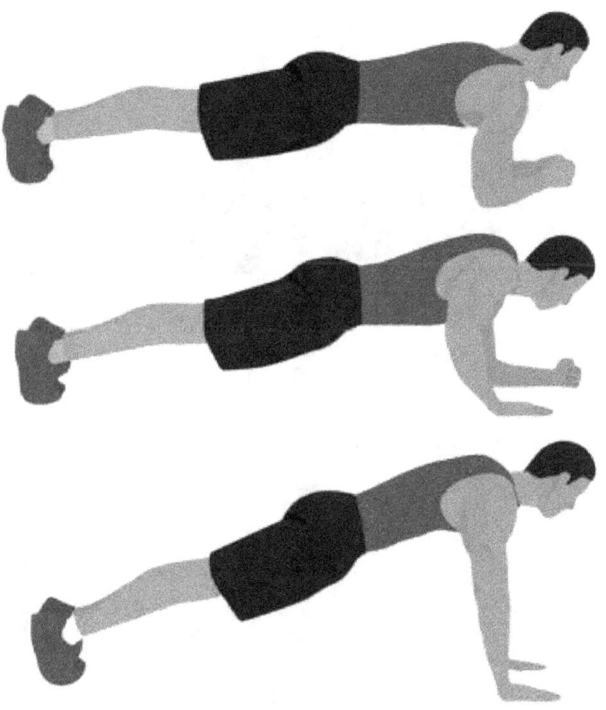

INSTRUCTIONS:

➤ Start this exercise in a plank position with your hands directly under your shoulders.

➤ Lower onto your forearms one arm at a time, then rise back to plank position one arm at a time.

➤ Aim for 20-30 seconds, gradually increasing to 45-60 seconds.

HOLLOW BODY HOLD

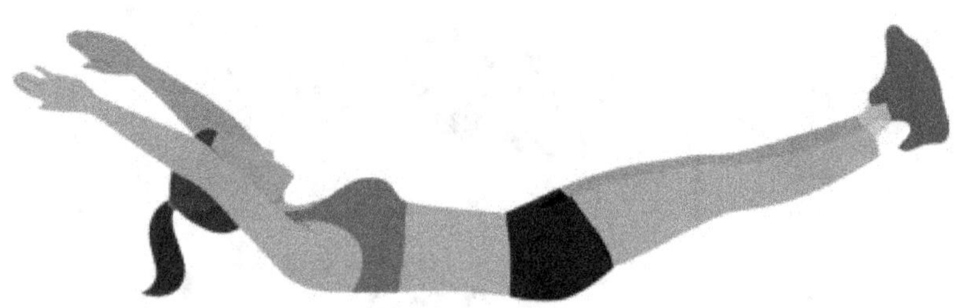

INSTRUCTIONS:

➢ Lie on your back and lift your shoulder blades and legs off the ground, creating a "hollow" shape with your body.

➢ Hold for 20-30 seconds to start, gradually increasing to 45-60 seconds.

WOODCHOPPERS

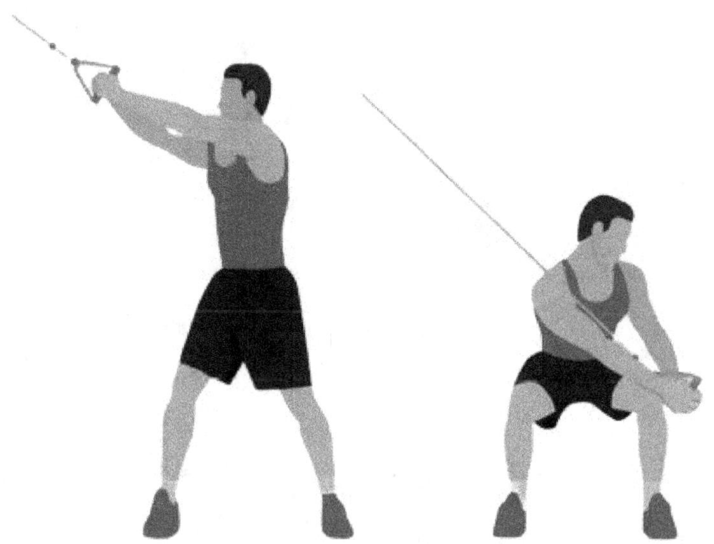

INSTRUCTIONS:

➢ Begin woodchoppers by standing with your feet shoulder-width apart, holding a weight or medicine ball with both hands.

➢ Rotate your torso and raise the weight diagonally across your body, then return to the starting position.

➢ Aim for 10-12 repetitions on each side to start, gradually increasing to 15-20 repetitions.

PILATES HUNDRED

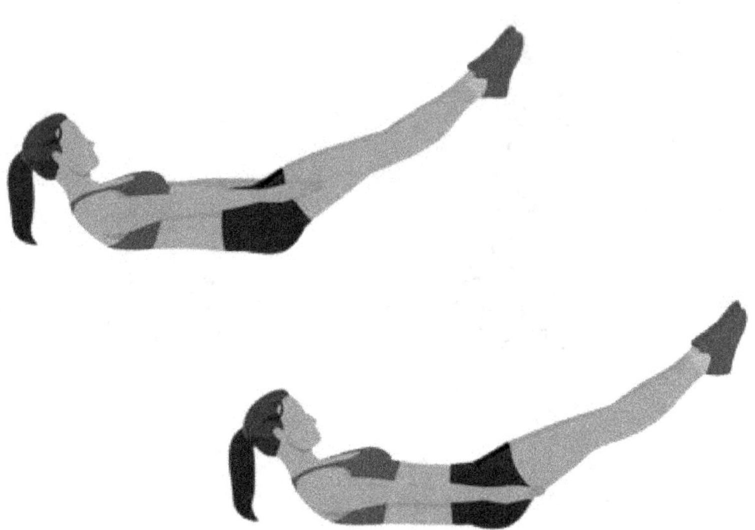

INSTRUCTIONS:

➢ Lie on your back with legs raised and arms by your sides.

➢ Next, gently lift your head, neck, and shoulders off the ground and pump your arms up and down.

➢ Aim for 10-15 seconds to start, gradually working up to 60 seconds.

HEEL TOUCHES

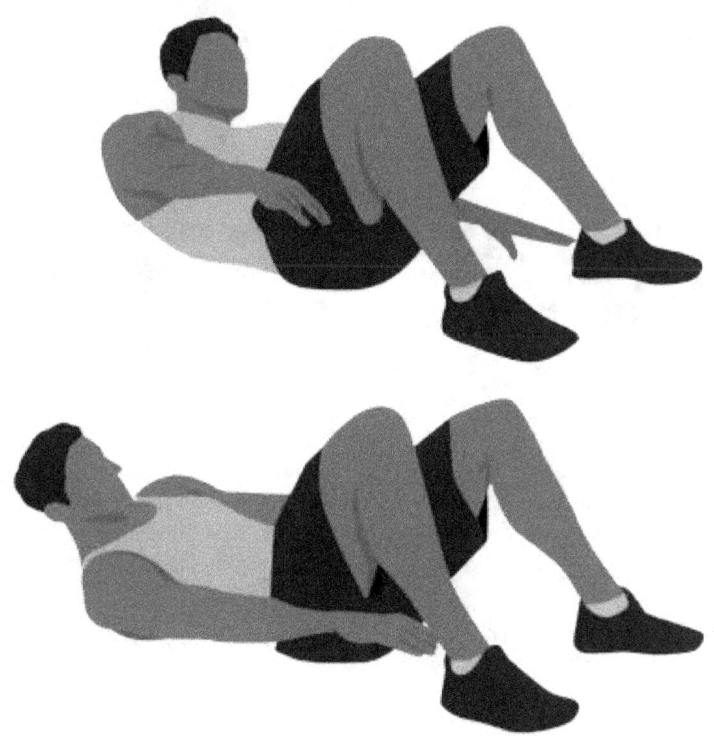

INSTRUCTIONS:

➢ Start this Heel Touches exercise by lying on your back with your knees bent and feet flat on the floor.

➢ Next, lift your shoulder blades off the ground and reach towards your heels, twisting your torso.

➢ Aim for 12-15 repetitions on each side.

KNEE TUCKS

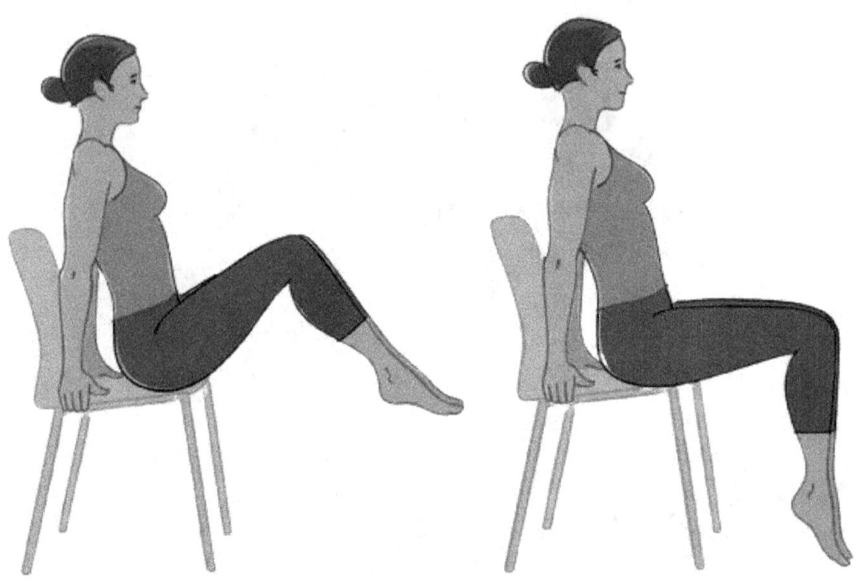

INSTRUCTIONS:

➤ Begin the Knee Tucks exercise by sitting on the edge of a chair/floor with your hands gripping the sides for support.

➤ Lift your knees towards your chest, then extend your legs back down.

➤ Aim for 10-12 repetitions to start, gradually increasing to 15-20 as strength improves.

OBLIQUE CRUNCHES

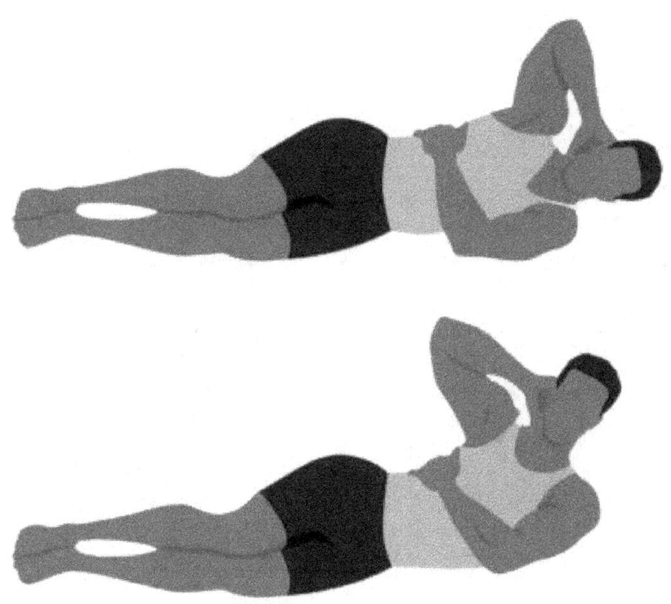

INSTRUCTIONS:

➤ Start the Oblique Crunches by lying on your side with knees bent and feet flat on the floor.

➤ Place your hands behind your head and lift your shoulder blades off the ground, twisting to touch your right elbow to your left knee, then alternating.

➤ Aim for 10-15 repetitions on each side to start, gradually increasing to 20-25 repetitions.

SEATED LEG LIFTS

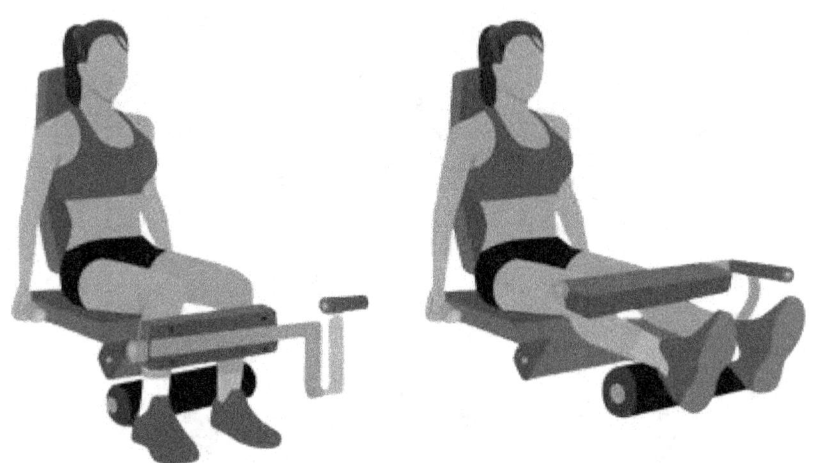

INSTRUCTIONS:

➤ Sit on the edge of a chair with your hands holding the sides for support.

➤ Lift your legs straight out in front of you, then lower them back down without touching the ground.

➤ Aim for 10-12 repetitions to start, gradually increasing to 15-20 as strength improves.

SEATED RUSSIAN TWISTS

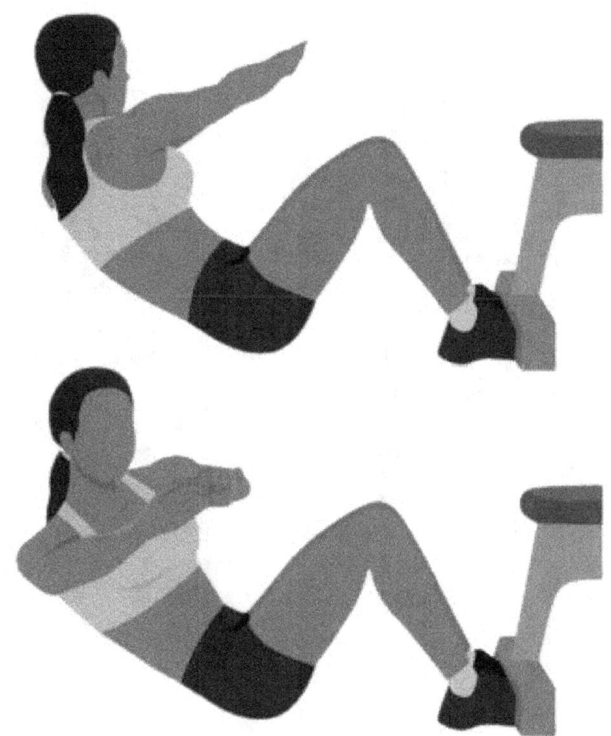

INSTRUCTIONS:

- ➢ Firstly, sit on the floor with your knees bent and feet flat.

- ➢ Next, lean back slightly and clasp your hands, then twist your torso from side to side.

- ➢ Aim for 10-12 repetitions on each side to start, gradually increasing to 15-20 repetitions.

CHAIR SIT-UPS

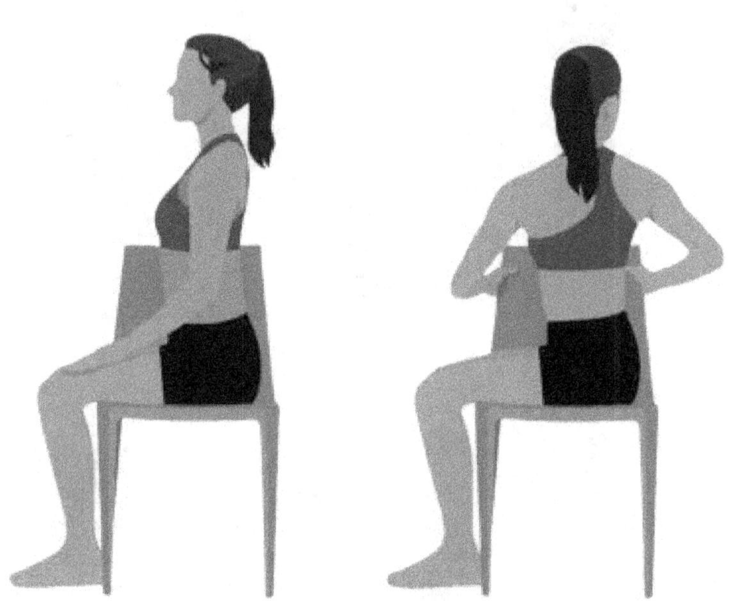

INSTRUCTIONS:

➢ Begin the Chair Sit-ups by sitting on the edge of a chair with your hands behind your head.

➢ Engage your core and lean back, then sit back up to perform a sit-up.

➢ Aim for 10-15 repetitions to start, gradually increasing to 20-25 as strength improves.

JACKKNIFE SIT-UP

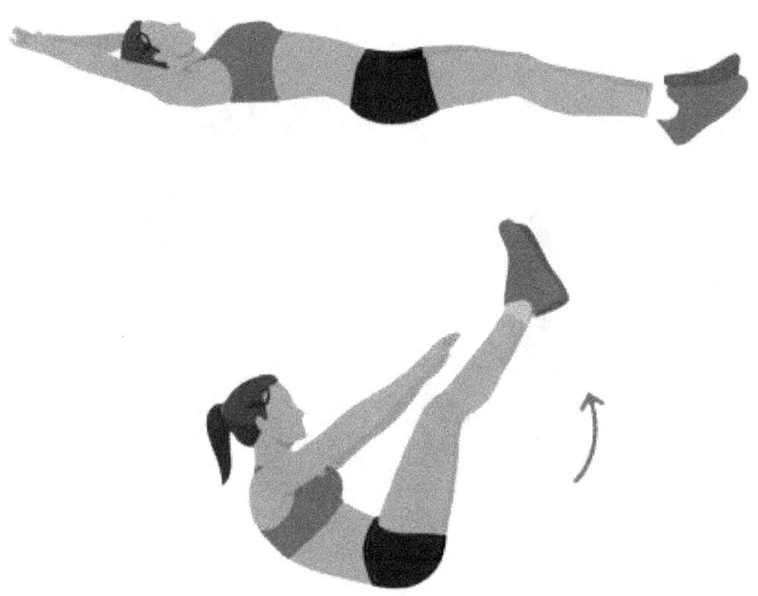

INSTRUCTIONS:

➢ Lie on your back with your legs extended and arms stretched overhead.

➢ Sit up, bringing your legs and arms to meet in the middle, then return to the starting position.

➢ Aim for 10-12 repetitions to start, gradually increasing to 15-20 as strength improves.

BEAR CRAWL

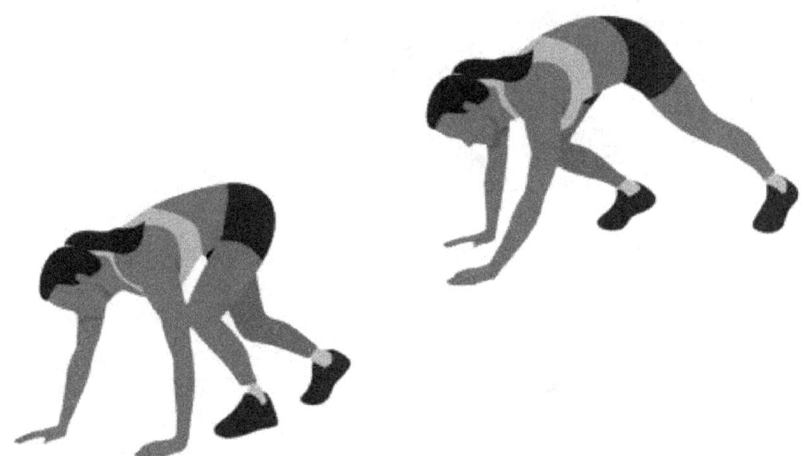

INSTRUCTIONS:

- ➢ Start on all fours, then lift your knees off the ground to hover.
- ➢ Crawl forward by moving opposite hand and foot together, then alternate.
- ➢ Aim for 20-30 seconds, gradually increasing to 45-60 seconds.

SPIDERMAN PLANK

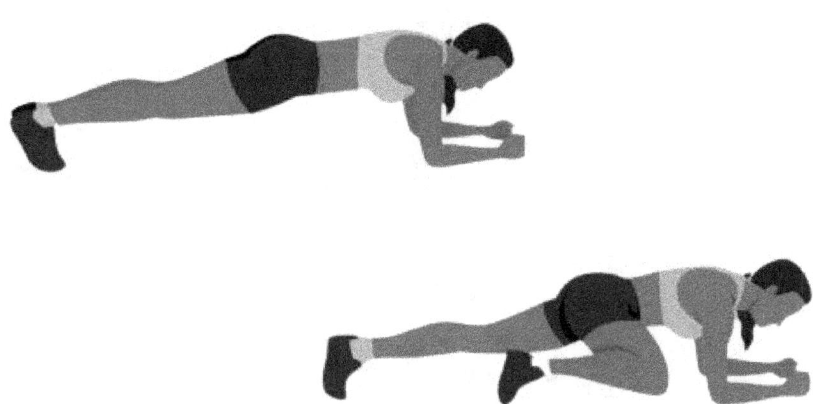

INSTRUCTIONS:

> Begin in a forearm plank position.

> Next, gently bring your right knee towards your right elbow, then return to the plank position.

> Repeat on the left side.

> Aim for 10-12 repetitions on each side to start, gradually increasing to 15-20 repetitions.

LEG CIRCLES

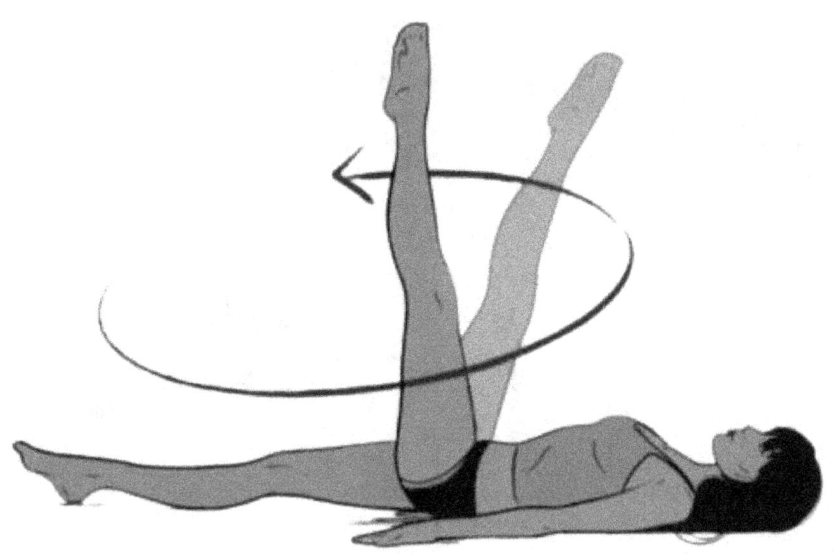

INSTRUCTIONS:

➢ Start this exercise by lying on your back with your legs extended.

➢ Lift one leg and make circular motions with it, clockwise and counterclockwise.

➢ Aim for 8-12 circles in each direction, then switch legs.

SIDE LYING LEG LIFTS

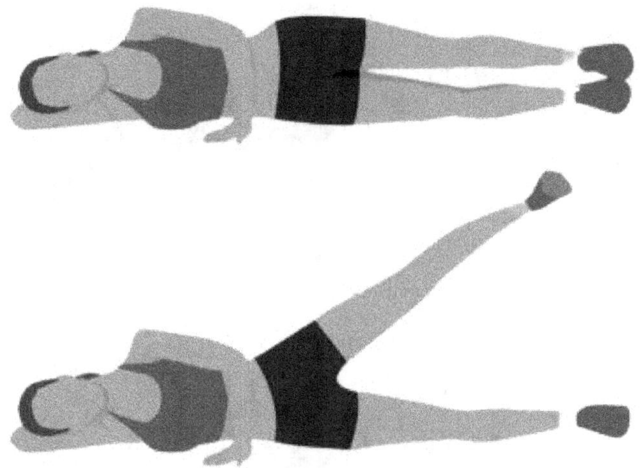

INSTRUCTIONS:

➢ Begin this core exercise by lying on your side with legs extended.

➢ Lift the top leg towards the ceiling, then lower back down.

➢ Aim for 10-12 repetitions on each side to start, gradually increasing to 15-20 repetitions.

SIDE PLANK LEG LIFTS

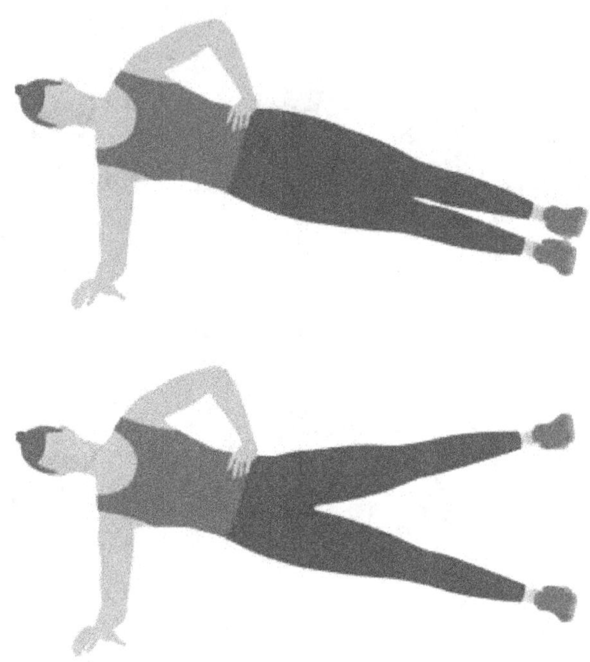

INSTRUCTIONS:

➤ Start in a side plank position with your body in a straight line.

➤ Next, gently lift your top leg towards the ceiling, then lower it back down.

➤ Aim for 10-12 repetitions on each side to start, gradually increasing to 15-20 repetitions.

PLANK WITH LEG LIFT

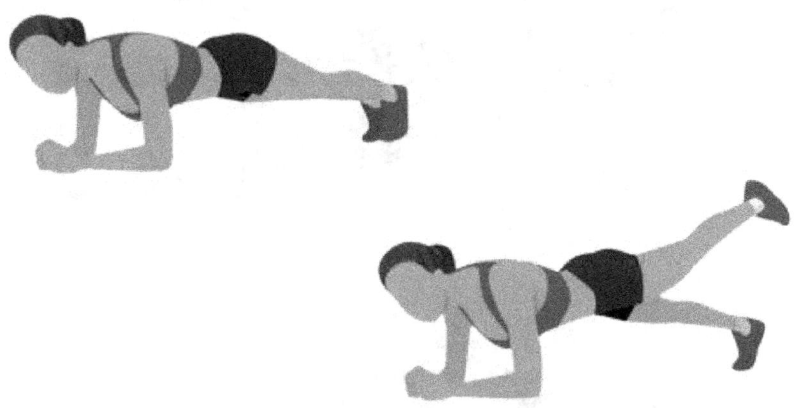

INSTRUCTIONS:

➢ Start in a forearm plank position.

➢ Lift one leg off the ground, hold it for a few seconds, then switch legs.

➢ Aim for 8-10 lifts on each leg.

SIDE PLANK CRUNCH

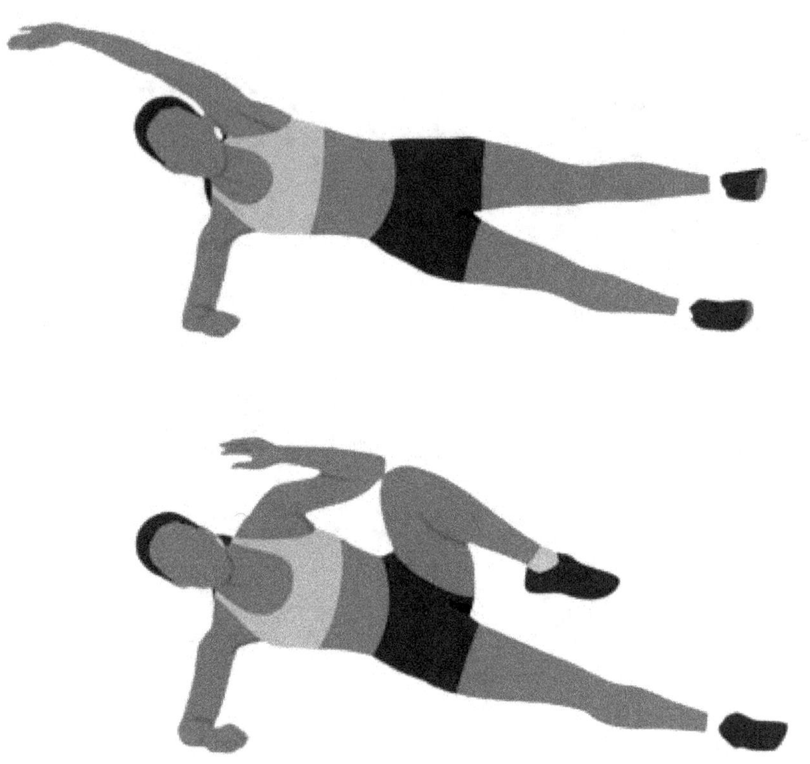

INSTRUCTIONS:

➢ Start in a side plank position with your body in a straight line.

➢ Bring your top elbow and top knee towards each other, then return to the starting position.

➢ Aim for 10-12 repetitions on each side to start, gradually increasing to 15-20 repetitions.

IN AND OUT ABS

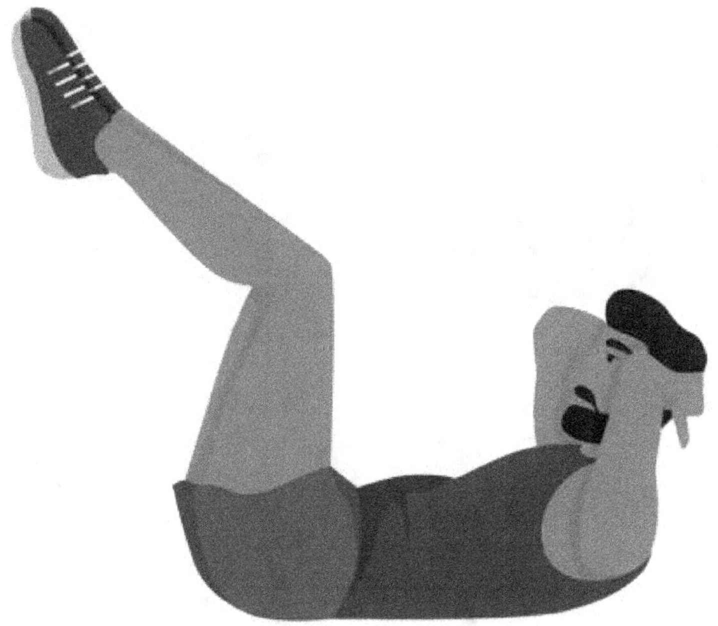

INSTRUCTIONS:

➢ Start this In and Out Abs exercise by sitting on the floor with your knees bent, and lean back slightly.

➢ Bring your knees towards your chest, then straighten your legs out in front of you.

➢ Aim for 15-20 repetitions to start, gradually increasing to 25-30 as strength improves.

SINGLE LEG STRETCH

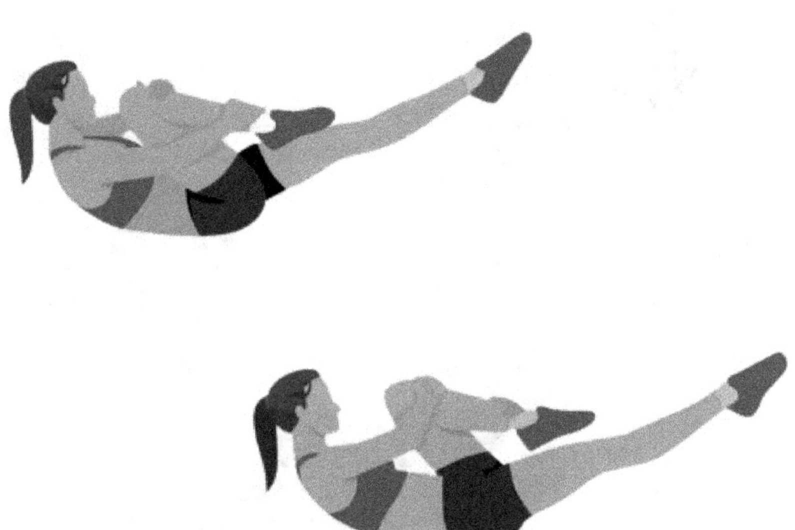

INSTRUCTIONS:

➢ Begin this exercise by lying on your back with your knees bent and shins parallel to the floor.

➢ Bring one knee towards your chest while extending the other leg, then switch.

➢ Aim for 12-15 repetitions on each side to start, gradually increasing to 20-25 repetitions.

CORKSCREW

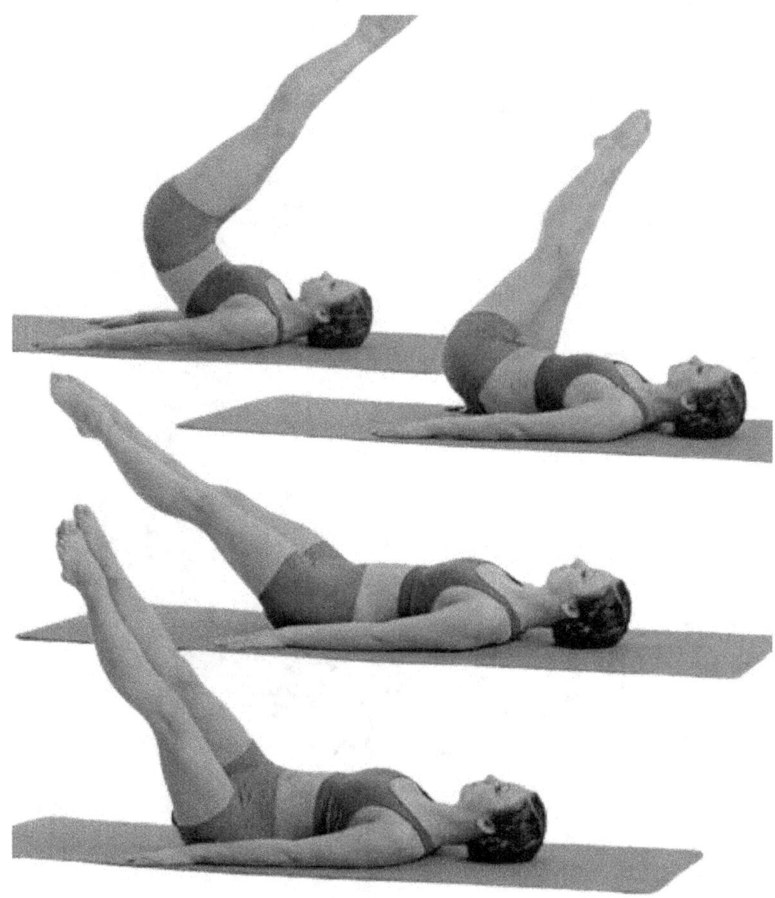

INSTRUCTIONS:

➢ Begin this Corkscrew exercise by lying on your back and extending your legs vertically towards the ceiling.

➢ Keeping your legs straight, lower them to one side in a circular motion, then bring them back up to the center and lower to the other side.

➢ Aim for 8-10 full circles.

PRONE COBRA

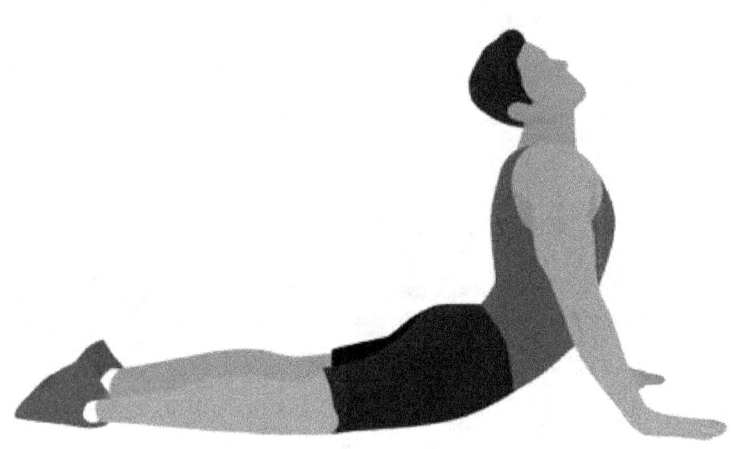

INSTRUCTIONS:

➢ Begin this Prone Cobra by lying on your stomach with your hands under your shoulders.

➢ Press through your hands to lift your chest off the ground, keeping your gaze forward.

➤ Hold for 15-20 seconds to start, gradually increasing to 30-45 seconds.

TRIANGLE POSE

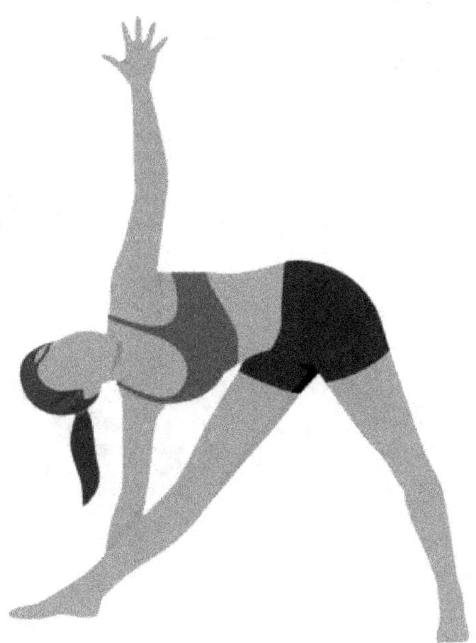

INSTRUCTIONS:

➤ Stand with your feet wide apart, one foot pointing forward and the other at a 90-degree angle.

➤ Reach towards the forward foot with your same-side arm, extending the opposite arm towards the ceiling.

➤ Hold for 20-30 seconds on each side.

TABLETOP

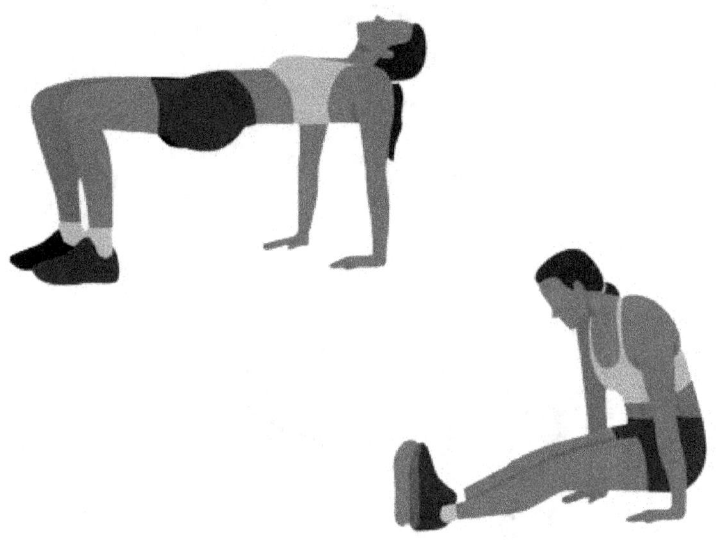

INSTRUCTIONS:

➢ Sit on the floor with your knees bent and hands placed behind you, fingers pointing towards your body.

➢ Lift your hips towards the ceiling, creating a tabletop position with your body.

➢ Hold for 20-30 seconds to start, gradually increasing to 45-60 seconds.

STANDING SIDE BEND

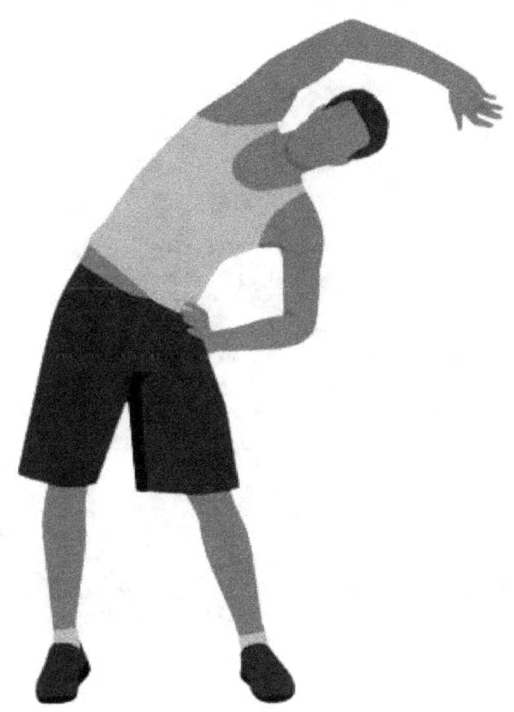

INSTRUCTIONS:

➢ Begin this core exercise by standing with your feet hip-width apart and arms by your sides.

➢ Next, raise one arm overhead and gently lean to the opposite side.

➢ Hold for 20-30 seconds on each side.

MERMAID

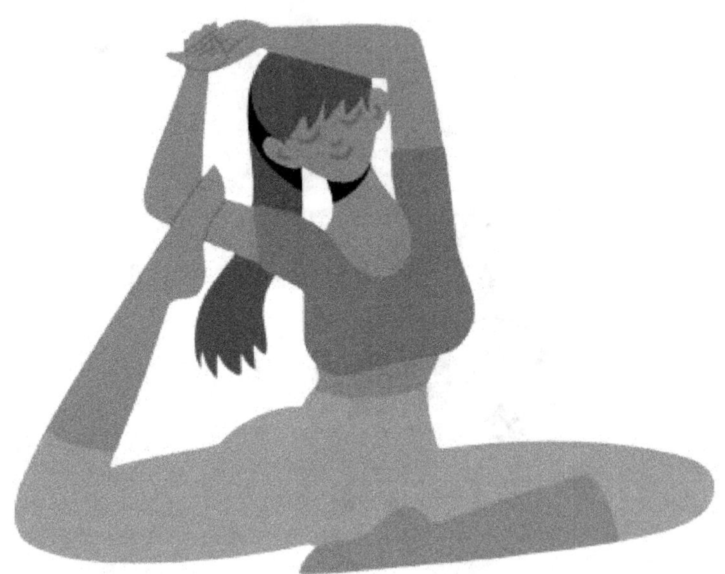

INSTRUCTIONS:

- ➤ Sit on the floor with your legs bent to one side, one hand on the floor for support.
- ➤ Extend your opposite arm overhead, then laterally bend towards the floor.
- ➤ Hold for 20-30 seconds on each side.

QUADRUPED

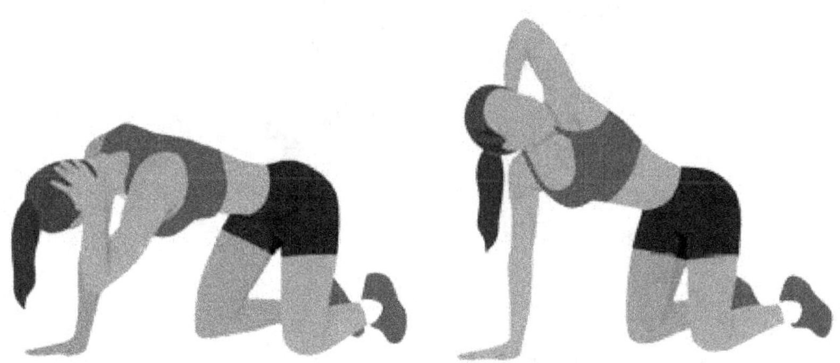

INSTRUCTIONS:

- ➤ Start on your hands and knees, with your wrists directly under your shoulders and knees under your hips.
- ➤ Engage your core and extend one arm and the opposite leg, then switch sides.
- ➤ Aim for 10-13 repetitions on each side.

CAT-COW

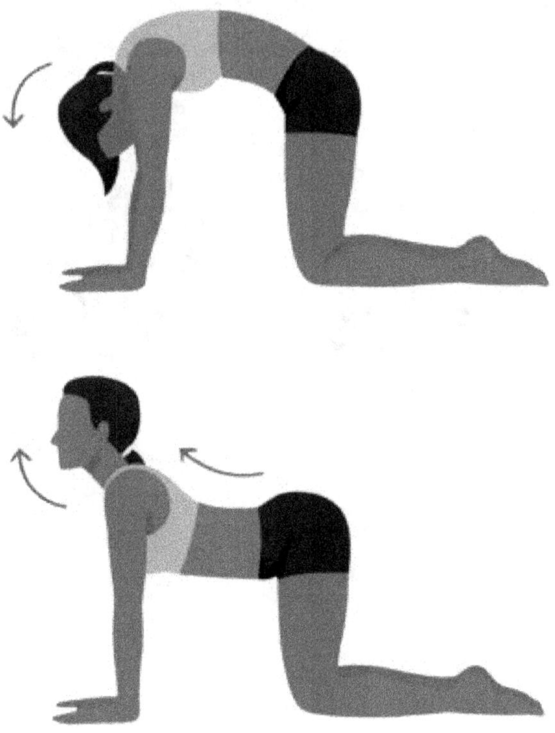

INSTRUCTIONS:

➢ Start on your hands and knees, with your wrists directly under your shoulders and knees under your hips.

➢ Arch your back upwards like an angry cat, then lower your back and lift your head, creating a cow-like shape.

➢ Move between these positions for 8-10 repetitions.

BOAT TWIST

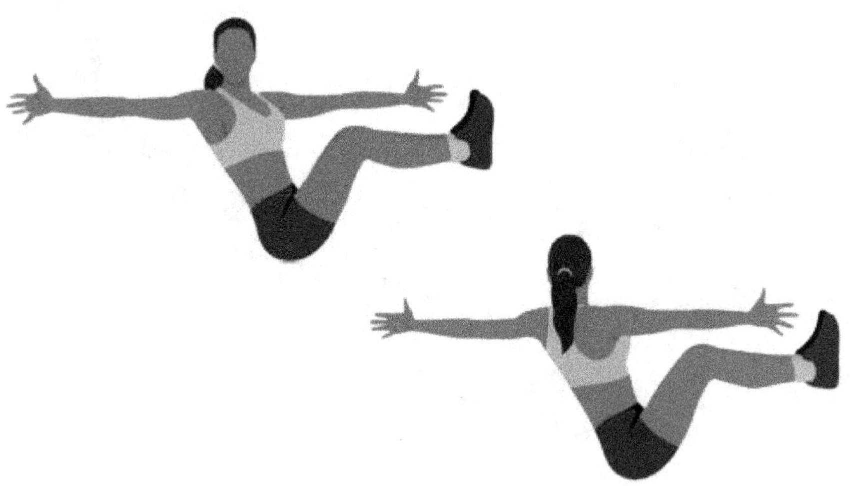

INSTRUCTIONS:

- ➢ Sit on the floor with your knees bent and lean back slightly, lifting your feet off the ground.
- ➢ Twist your torso from side to side.
- ➢ Aim for 12-16 twists on each side.

PILATES TEASER

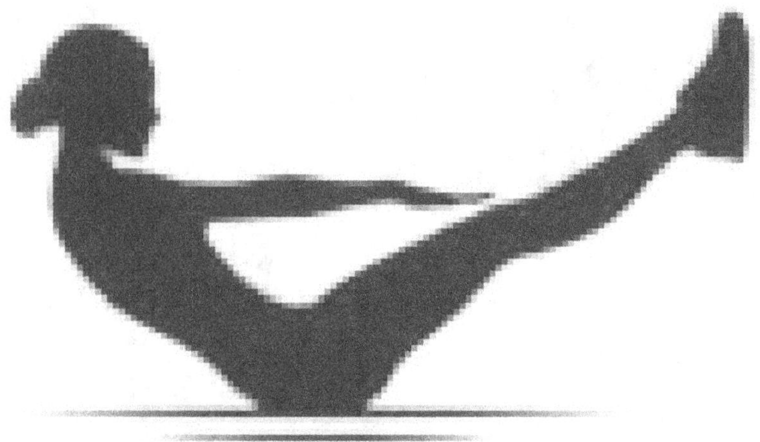

INSTRUCTIONS:

➤ Start lying on your back with your legs extended and arms reaching overhead.

➤ Lift your legs, arms, and head, and roll up to a seated position, then roll back down.

➤ Aim for 8-10 repetitions.

ERIC A. RANDELL

30-DAY

CORE EXERCISE CHALLENGE FOR SENIORS OVER 50

DAY	1ST EXERCISE	2ND EXERCISE	3RD EXERCISE
1	30 seconds plank	15 Russian twists on each side	10 dead bugs on each side
2	45 seconds bridge	20 tuck crunches	12 leg raises
3	1-minute boat pose	30 bicycle crunches	15 second plank on each side
4	40 seconds Superman	20 flutter kicks	12 bird dogs on each side
5	1-minute side plank (30 seconds on each side)	20 sit-ups	12 bird dogs on each side

DAY	1ST EXERCISE	2ND EXERCISE	3RD EXERCISE
6	REST	REST	REST
7	45-second plank	25 V-sit	15 stability ball crunches
8	1-minute plank	30 side plank leg lifts (15 on each side)	20 Russian twists
9	1-minute bridge	40 bicycle crunches	15 scissor kicks
10	1-minute boat pose	40 mountain climbers	20 tuck crunches

DAY	1ST EXERCISE	2ND EXERCISE	3RD EXERCISE
11	1-minute Superman	25 leg raises	15 bird dogs on each side
12	1-minute side plank (30 seconds on each side)	20 sit-ups	12 leg raises
13	REST	REST	REST
14	1-minute plank	35 V-sit	20 stability ball crunches
15	1-minute plank with leg lift	30 Russian twists	20 bicycle crunches

DAY	1ST EXERCISE	2ND EXERCISE	3RD EXERCISE
16	1-minute hollow body hold	35 flutter kicks	20 bear crawls
17	1-minute boat pose	40 mountain climbers	25 tuck crunches
18	1-minute side plank (30 seconds on each side)	25 side plank leg lifts (15 on each side))	20 scissor kicks
19	1-minute Russian twists	35 V-sit	20 reverse crunches
20	REST	REST	REST

DAY	1ST EXERCISE	2ND EXERCISE	3RD EXERCISE
21	1.5-minute plank	40 stability ball crunches	30 bicycle crunches
22	1.5-minute plank	40 scissor kicks	25 Russian twists
23	1.5-minute boat pose	50 mountain climbers	30 tuck crunches
24	1.5-minute side plank (45 seconds on each side)	30 leg raises	20 bear crawls
25	2-minute plank	40 V-sit	25 stability ball crunches

DAY	1ST EXERCISE	2ND EXERCISE	3RD EXERCISE
26	1.5-minute Russian twists	45 bicycle crunches	25 scissor kicks
27	REST	REST	REST
28	2-minute plank	50 mountain climbers	35 Russian twists
29	2-minute plank	40 leg raises	30 stability ball crunches
30	2.5-minute plank	50 V-sit	40 Russian twists

Weekly Exercise Planner

WEEKS	1ST EXERCISE	2ND EXERCISE	3RD EXERCISE
MON			
TUE			
WED			
THU			
FRI			
SAT			
SUN			

Weekly Exercise Planner

WEEKS	1ST EXERCISE	2ND EXERCISE	3RD EXERCISE
MON			
TUE			
WED			
THU			
FRI			
SAT			
SUN			

Weekly Exercise Planner

WEEKS	1ST EXERCISE	2ND EXERCISE	3RD EXERCISE
MON			
TUE			
WED			
THU			
FRI			
SAT			
SUN			

Weekly Exercise Planner

WEEKS	1ST EXERCISE	2ND EXERCISE	3RD EXERCISE
MON			
TUE			
WED			
THU			
FRI			
SAT			
SUN			

Weekly Exercise Planner

WEEKS	1ST EXERCISE	2ND EXERCISE	3RD EXERCISE
MON			
TUE			
WED			
THU			
FRI			
SAT			
SUN			

Weekly Exercise Planner

WEEKS	1ST EXERCISE	2ND EXERCISE	3RD EXERCISE
MON			
TUE			
WED			
THU			
FRI			
SAT			
SUN			

NOTES

NOTES

NOTES

NOTES

NOTES

NOTES

NOTES

NOTES

NOTES

NOTES

NOTES

www.ingramcontent.com/pod-product-compliance
Lightning Source LLC
Chambersburg PA
CBHW050832260726
48660CB00006B/2196